INFERTILITY

INFERTILITY

The silent and unseen issue

A resource from Mission to Marriage
& Christian Marriage Ministries

Rosemary and Barry Jubraj

With a preface by John Wyatt,
Professor of Neonatal Paediatrics,
University College, London

RoperPenberthy Publishing Ltd
Horsham, England

First Published by Mission to Marriage. Reg Charity No. 273658.
Registered office and address for correspondence:
Allt Goch, Penegoes, Machynlleth, Powys, SY20 8UW
www.christianmarriageministries.co.uk

British Library Cataloguing in Publication data
A catalogue record for this book is available from the
British Library.

ISBN 978-1-903905-31-9

Any profits from this book will be used for ministry purposes by the charity. The charity would like to emphasise that the writers have asked to forgo any royalties to support the work of Mission to Marriage & Christian Marriage Ministries, an offer we accept with gratitude.

Cover illustration by Sue Stamper-Iveson.

Designed and produced by RoperPenberthy Publishing Ltd,
Horsham, West Sussex.

Typeset by Avocet Typeset, Chilton, Aylesbury, Bucks
Printed and bound by J. H. Haynes & Co. Ltd, Sparkford

Contents

Commendations

Barry and Rosemary open their hearts in this book, which could be a great encouragement to other couples, like themselves, struggling with infertility. I remember well how bleak those words sounded – 'infertile', 'infertility' – when my wife and I were struggling with the same issues. They felt like a prison door slamming shut. How I wish that we had had Rosemary and Barry's readiness to look deep into their hearts, and to open their pain fully to each other. Now in this book they do the same for others facing childlessness, and I know that this painful but sensible guide could bring encouragement and support to many.

Steve Motyer, Theology and Counselling Course Leader,
London School of Theology.

The wisdom in this book came at a great price. Barry and Rosemary have displayed real emotional courage, as they open their hearts and their Bibles to tackle this widespread but so often silent and unseen issue of infertility. I am convinced this is not just a book that will be a great help to couples facing the heartbreak of infertility, but a must-read for those involved in caring for the church family.

Rico Tice, Associate Minister (Evangelism),
All Souls Church, Langham Place, London.

The style of the book has a warmth and supportive feel which works well for this tough subject. Barry and Rosemary have clearly worked through so many of the issues and have an ability to express them accessibly for others.

The topics are dealt with honestly with a helpful analysis of the different stages in dealing with the reality and the grief. The frequent reminder that everyone is different is essential to counter the tendency to look for quick solutions to alleviate pain. The section on 'Identity' is such a crucial one and confronts the difficulty of 'reaching for the invisible God' in the turmoil of emotional crisis. At these times God so often feels very distant and they recognise that this only adds to the blame and despair. The biblical material gives a helpful framework for the Christian living in a fallen world.

There are no easy answers to this and other painful issues of life. But we have a God who is compassionate and in his providence has a place of service in his kingdom for each of us. I was glad to see this message of encouragement within the book. The section on moving forward and practical care of yourselves is a helpful round-up of the book's main themes.

Sheena Gilles, Formerly on the senior pastoral staff of All Souls Church, Langham Place, London, and of Duke Street Church, Richmond.

Preface

Infertility is a silent and devastating sorrow which affects about one in six of all couples in our society. Yet the pain of childlessness is rarely acknowledged. It's possible for churches and for Christian people to seem insensitive and heedless of the hidden grief which many childless people experience. In my work as a paediatrician and Christian ethicist I have had the privilege of sharing the struggles and questions of many couples faced with the painful dilemmas which infertility poses.

Rosemary and Barry Jubraj are uniquely qualified to provide this unusual and practical resource for couples facing infertility. Both of them are qualified health professionals who have undertaken further theological training. Both of them have years of practical experience providing pastoral support within the church family and Barry is currently training as a Christian counsellor.

It's been a privilege for me to share their journey through infertility over a number of years, and I have admired and respected their honesty, openness and commitment in struggling to find God's way for them as a couple. This book is born from Rosemary and Barry's own experience and gives an honest and realistic account of their feelings and responses, together with thoughtful reflections from the framework of their biblical Christian worldview. Like the Psalmist they don't hesitate from expressing their negative emotions to God and I suspect there are many couples who will find their own unspoken feelings mirrored in these pages. Each chapter ends with practical exercises and suggestions for personal reflection, discussion and action, together with down-to-earth guidance on ways of moving forward through the pain towards acceptance and healing.

This remarkable book provides a valuable resource, not only for couples facing the pain and uncertainty of childlessness, but also for all those who seek to support them in their journey.

John Wyatt
Professor of Neonatal Paediatrics
University College London

Prologue

We would like to introduce this resource about infertility with an account of Rosemary's personal experience of trying to come to terms with the news of infertility when it was new. This account was written some years ago.

The pain of childlessness should never be underestimated.

Barry and I had been married for five years and had been trying for a family for two years. We had been subjected to numerous tests to establish a possible reason for our infertility. Some of these were painful and humiliating. However, I found the worst pain came each time with the results. After each test I actually prayed that the doctors would find something wrong, which may sound a bit crazy. I wanted to find a reason for our infertility – some scientific basis. I am a logical person who usually takes a methodical approach to problem-solving. This then compounded my pain when the doctors could find nothing wrong with either of us in the first few months of testing – I had no reason, other than to trust that God had a reason.

At one point Barry explained that he believed that God was stopping us from having children. He must be right, as there appears to be no earthly reason why we shouldn't conceive, therefore there must be a heavenly one. This is still sinking into my consciousness at the moment, and it's a tough one as I know that I should seek and obey God's will for us. When his will seems to be saying quite clearly 'no children at the moment, possibly never' that's a hard thing to hear and accept.

Being told by our consultant gynaecologist to relax, take six months off from trying to conceive and not think about children was one of the hardest things said to me. She did not say this in a dispassionate way, but I feel did show some significant lack of insight into what it's like waiting to conceive. (My consultant is a parent.) No one, other than other infertile couples, can understand what it's like. I find it impossible not to think about hoping for a child. When I try not to think about it I am making a conscious decision not to, which makes me think about what I am trying not to think about! I am also surrounded by constant reminders – family and friends have children from whom I have no desire to disconnect myself. Some of these are the very people who support me most by allowing me to be me. Everywhere I go I see children, I see heavily pregnant women, I even see baby clothes in Mothercare. Yes, just walking past a shop with things for babies hurts; another reminder of my situation.

Each month my body reminds me that I am a woman, designed to carry children. I have come to hate period pain, not only for the way it makes me feel physically, but also the stark reminder that once again I have come through a cycle without getting pregnant. My hormones seem to scream at me.

After two years of trying we were offered IVF by our consultant. After a great deal of thought and prayer we decided not to try conceiving in this way. This is a complex issue and we did not take our decision lightly. There is no right or wrong answer, unfortunately the Bible does not have any clear guidance on this so we asked a lot of questions, prayed about it and just tried to listen to what God was saying to us. It was a really tough decision to make.

I feel that I spend my life on an emotional roller coaster. After each period has finished I have about two weeks in each month when I feel positive. I think 'maybe I'm pregnant this month'. I am a naturally optimistic person, so I find it easy to think positively. Then the hormones kick in and I start feeling pre-menstrual. At this point my emotions take a nose-dive as I feel fragile due to PMT and the reality hits that I'm not pregnant. Then my period starts, I feel lousy from the pain and know for sure that I'm not pregnant. Another month gone. Over the last two years it has taken longer for my emotions to start the climb uphill again. Regular disappointment takes its toll. There have been times when I've felt so low, crying, wanting to hit something, that I've started to wonder if I'm actually losing my mind. I can tell everything to Barry, even these fears, which is vital as he can reassure me that I am not going mad and that it's OK to cry. You would think one way of counteracting such fears is to immerse oneself in other activities and not give oneself too much time to dwell on the situation. I have always led a busy life, none more so than of late. I work full time, enjoy a busy social life with friends and family, am involved in areas of service at church and have even taken up a new hobby. All of these I enjoy immensely, and yet my desire for children is always there.

I don't feel like a biological failure, I just feel incomplete as a woman. There is a song we sing at church about being complete in God's grace. I find this hard to sing as I know I should feel complete through my salvation in Christ. It's one of those head versus heart things. I know the theory of grace and of being complete in God; however I find it hard to feel it in my life at this time.

I have a close relationship with my two young nephews, which I have worked hard to foster, not only because I love them dearly as part of the family, but also because I have come to realise they may be the children I can be closest to in my life. I take time off work to spend quality time with them, and my heart leaps when I walk into the room to be greeted by a smile and a hug from them. And yet, when one of them falls over and bumps themselves, even if their special auntie is with them, the only person they want to be comforted by is mummy. I yearn to be that person for a child. It hurts when my nephews run past me to my sister – though of course this is exactly how it should be. I don't want them to run to me, I want my own children to run to me.

I don't ever want to stop spending time with my nephews; whenever I have seen them I usually feel emotionally fragile for a couple of days afterwards. This is because they mean so much to me and I miss them dreadfully.

There is a great temptation to put one's life on hold whilst waiting and hoping for a child. Barry and I have worked hard at not doing this by continuing to plan holidays abroad and pursuing activities that would otherwise be precluded by pregnancy and young children. We do this on the basis that if I do fall pregnant any of these things can be cancelled for something of infinitely greater importance.

I am a naturally chatty person who enjoys a good natter pretty much any time of the day. However, I have found our infertility a hard thing to talk about – both to God and other people. I find it difficult to say things out loud that are painful for me to hear. I have managed to talk things through with some of my family and a few close friends who are sensitive enough to know never to ask me how I feel but are always willing to listen when I need to talk. This means I am in control of when I want to talk, which is important for me. I'm not good at being caught off guard.

It was after a year of trying to conceive that I found myself chatting to a friend. She happened to be with me when I was feeling particularly low and we just got talking, I don't know why but I just felt that I could trust her. After pouring out a lot of what was on my mind she explained her situation and we found that we had a lot in common. She could identify directly with all the things I was saying, especially how I felt so isolated at times. I am deeply thankful to God for leading us to one another as she has been able to provide me with a great deal of empathetic support. Whenever I spend time with her I always come away realising afresh that I am not alone in what I am going through. Finding someone else to talk to who has been through similar experiences is invaluable. My friend has often reflected that she can now see a reason for all that she went through as she has been able to offer me such support. Maybe this is God's plan for me – to be able to use my experiences to help others.

I have been surprised by the thoughtlessness of some people who have the temerity to ask us if we want children or if we have them – and then look me in the eye and advise me not to leave it too long. People so often assume that all Christian married couples want children and can have children. The people who ask me are the very people with whom I most vehemently do not want to share my situation. How dare they suggest how I should live my life! It feels as if they are criticising me for not yet perpetuating the human race. Now of course I never let on how they make me feel – yet part of me wishes I could, not in an unkind way, just a way that would help stop them saying something similar to someone else. Barry is better at dealing with such comments than I am. He has been known to reply, 'How do you know we can have children?' – which usually stops people in their tracks. He doesn't do that if I'm there as he knows I want to retain my composure and for me to hear a direct challenge like that would probably make me cry.

I find it hard to trust God for my future – particularly with respect to what job I will do. I am not a career woman; I have actually left the profession that could have offered a career path three years ago, one year before starting to try for a family. In the back of my mind I always thought I would give up work to have a family – I wasn't anticipating working right through to retirement.

This is one situation in my life over which I have absolutely no control. I'm not a control freak, however I like things to be organised and have a handle on what's going on. The thing that helps me most to cope is the assurance that God is in control. I have to keep in mind how else he may be able to use me in his service without children.

I don't think my desire for children will ever stop; certainly not during my child-bearing years. However I hope I can accept God's calling for me at this time with patience and trust.

Welcome and Introduction

Infertility has placed an enormous pressure on our marriage. We have made mistakes in handling the issues associated with infertility, but since we know that God's desire is for Christians to remain within their marriages (1 Corinthians 7), we have worked hard in God's strength to rescue and sustain our marriage. During this process we have grown both as individuals and in our understanding of God. Our desire is to help you think through the issues around infertility that affect *your* marriage.

Overall aims of this infertility resource:

- To promote discussion within your own marriage, particularly with respect to infertility issues.
- To explore what the Bible says about children and how our faith as Christians can help us to move forward in spite of infertility.
- To consider how to face the future with your spouse when faced with infertility.

How the resource works

You will see from the first aim that we want you to talk with one another openly and honestly. This is a key part of the Christian Marriage Ministries ethos.

To facilitate your discussion, we will be sharing our story of infertility. This will illustrate how some of the issues around infertility can affect us and our marriages. We will also use the Bible to gain insight into God's perspective on infertility. There will be relevant questions for you to consider for yourselves as individuals and as a couple.

We suggest that you work through each chapter and reflect upon the material. The questions at the end will work best if each of you looks at them separately, writing down your thoughts. We then suggest that you come back together to discuss your thoughts and try to apply the principles to your own marriage. In addition, we have included some creative ideas that may also help you explore the issues raised. You may be able to think of others.

We appreciate that your situation may feel very raw and you may not yet be ready to think about some or all of the questions. It is important to give yourselves time to process your situation. Don't attempt to move forward too soon, but don't put it off indefinitely either. If you are not ready yet, perhaps you could consider making a note to re-read the questions at a later date in order to see whether you would feel ready to have a go at thinking about them.

If you are helping an infertile couple

Our hope is that this resource will also be useful for helpers. The resource can help you act as a facilitator in promoting discussion within the marriage. We would recommend that you bear in mind that infertility causes unique pain and there is no similar life experience with which to compare. Reading through our story first may help you to gain some perspective on the issues involved.

What the resource will NOT do

It won't answer all your questions

- We don't claim to have all the answers to the tough questions that you may have about infertility. We ourselves are continuing to learn through the mistakes that we made in our own marriage as well as from the progress that God has granted us.

It won't provide a quick fix

- We have come to realise that there is no quick fix to a marriage affected by infertility, but our experience is that God has wonderfully ministered to and preserved us in spite of our pain. His work in us is a lifelong process.

It won't tell you what to do

- We won't be trying to tell you what to do; for example whether or not to pursue IVF, fostering or adoption. As such we won't give a detailed account here of our decision-making in these matters.[1]

We wish you peace and blessing as you use this resource.

[1] We would not wish to unduly influence other couples regarding whether or not to have fertility treatment, which is why we have not discussed the reasons for our decisions in this book. We were greatly helped in our thinking and decisions by Professor John Wyatt through chapter 3 of his book, *Matters of Life and Death*, Leicester, 1998.

1. Telling our story

a. Our background as individuals

Rosemary
I was brought up in a secure Christian home and had a stable childhood. I brought a sense of reserve from family life into adulthood. As a teenager, I never assumed that I would marry, but presumed that if I did, children would follow.

Barry
My family background was complex and turbulent at times, involving violence, parental separation, re-marriage and half-siblings. Whatever Christians may believe about the source of suffering, I feel that these circumstances were used by God to strengthen me in spite of frequent feelings of insecurity. I recall vowing as a child not to make the same mistakes as my parents if ever I married and became a parent. For many years I felt negative about marriage, not wanting to be hurt in ways that I had observed as a child. My view of fatherhood has since required some adjustment in the light of my experiences.

b. What happened to us as a married couple?

Given our individual backgrounds, we both came into our marriage in 1995 with the unconscious assumption that we would have children. We waited for three years before trying for a family, during which time we both had busy jobs, studies and church commitments. After six months of trying we consulted our GP and there was a time frame of about 18 months between our first GP consultation to the final meeting with a consultant about our infertility. This included us both having tests and a lot of time spent thinking that this would be unexplained infertility. It eventually transpired that Barry's hernia surgery in 1997 was the most likely cause. We felt some pressure from our consultant to have IVF but after much thought and prayer we decided not to do this. We also decided not to adopt or foster, which means that we remained childless.

During the period from starting to try for a family, through to our final decision about fertility treatment, we drifted apart in our marriage. Although infertility was the primary cause, experiencing burnout in our jobs and in our church commitments at the time made matters worse. We reached a crisis point where we were unable to communicate; and in spite of our Christian faith, we twice seriously contemplated separation. With God's help, our relationship has been rescued but it has been a long and painful journey towards restoration in our marriage and coming to terms with infertility. The journey continues to this day.

c. What principles does our story illustrate?

Hopes and expectations:

Many agree that each person brings hopes and expectations about marriage and family life from childhood into adulthood. Everyone is prone to making assumptions, although neither of us ever assumed that we would get married and have children. Perhaps marriage and family life seemed intangible or abstract to us as children and young people, which is understandable.

The impact of past experiences on the present:

Many psychologists and counsellors believe that whether we know it or not, past experiences contribute to the person that we are today. The crisis point in our marriage developed partly because of childhood influences that limited our ability to communicate about such a painful matter as our infertility. Barry's childhood insecurities and Rosemary's reserve could have been significant contributory factors.

Infertility is a pressure on marriage – but marriage can survive it

We have found that infertility put an enormous strain on our marriage, but not in isolation. Other areas of life such as work, church commitments and other relationships can add to the pressure. Chapter 5 of this book highlights some of the strategies that have helped us, in God's strength, to survive as a married couple in spite of infertility.

Infertility is a journey in our lives – and you are not alone!

Some friends who were also struggling with fertility issues introduced us to the concept of it being a journey. This describes the progression from hearing the news of infertility through discussing and choosing options, and trying to come to terms with the news as time progresses. It also describes how our relationships with God and each other change with time and the process of grief.

Like us, each of you as a couple will have your own story of infertility. You will also be at a different stage of your journey from other couples and from us. For some of you, your news might be new and very raw. Others of you may have known about your infertility for some time. Some of you may be considering or currently receiving IVF treatment, or you may be considering / trying for adoption.

Each of you will have different struggles, whether this be with yourself, your spouse, family, friends, work colleagues or with God. The struggle isn't helped by the lack of discussion about this subject. This may be partly because infertility is an unseen problem. If someone has a broken leg, this is visible and they clearly cannot walk. People are unlikely to ask the victim of a broken leg if they can walk! In contrast, infertility is invisible, but infertile couples may be asked, quite understandably, if they have children, which may lead to awkwardness. This may partly explain why coping with infertility is so hard.

Currently, approximately one in six couples in the UK experience difficulties in having children[2]. However, as this issue is not widely discussed, infertile couples may feel very isolated.

An openness to discussing infertility involves making yourselves vulnerable in many ways. However, we have found that God has placed people in our path as a couple, to accompany us on at least part of our journey. As we have become more open about our own infertility, we have encountered more and more couples in similar situations.

[2] Treasurer, British Fertility Society: Radio 5 Live Interview, August 2005

d. Timeline exercise and questions

Explanation

As you reflect on our story, it may remind you of your own childhood experiences and the impact on the present. Exploring this for yourself and as a couple can help you to understand each other better as you face the pain of infertility, whether it is new or long-standing.

Therefore, the aim of this exercise and the associated questions is to help you individually and as a couple to bring to mind events in your lives and to think about how they may influence your response to infertility.

How to do the exercise

Drawing the timeline and thinking about the questions should probably take a maximum of 45 minutes to an hour (30–45 minutes for the timeline and 15 minutes maximum for the questions); but may take less time depending on how much detail you wish to include in the timeline. Feel free to adapt the timeline method in any way that suits you in order to illustrate the events that you wish to record.

Timeline

Take a large sheet of paper and draw a straight line across it. Mark the start of the line with your date of birth. Then mark along the line events from your own life journey that are important to you. Events may include those that happened in the following periods of your life:

- *Childhood* (for example, moving house, starting school, exams, etc.)
- *Pre-marriage* (for example, leaving home, family deaths, work milestones, etc.)
- *Marriage* (for example, meeting your spouse, engagement dates, wedding date, moving house, etc.)
- *Infertility* (for example, when you started trying for children, significant medical test dates, news of a diagnosis, news of family or friends getting pregnant, making decisions about treatment, etc.)

Aim for 15–20 events on your timeline; but feel free to include more or less if you wish. When you have done this, please have a look at the following questions:

1. List a maximum of five hopes or expectations that you had about marriage and family as a child/young person. Go with your initial thoughts:

2. Using your timeline, how might your own childhood experiences have impacted your hopes, expectations and how you feel now? List your thoughts here:

When you have finished, come back together and talk each other through your timelines and responses. You may not feel able to discuss all of this at once in the time suggested. If this is the case, you may wish to take more time or schedule in a second discussion time.

2. Our responses to infertility, feelings and the effects

Each of us responds to difficult situations in different ways. In this section, we will describe how we felt and how we responded. The questions at the end will then help you to discuss your own responses with your spouse.

a. How did each of us respond?

Rosemary

I had made few assumptions about whether I would get married, but had the expectation that children would follow if I did. I was surprised at the intensity of the pain I experienced when it became clear that we may not have children. Feelings of isolation from Barry and friends/family who were having children were significant. At a conscious level there was no anger towards Barry in spite of the physical problem lying with him, but I was consciously angry towards God, although I found this enormously difficult to admit and express.

These feelings were very raw in the first few years. There were certain triggers (for example, hearing about friends falling pregnant, seeing newborn babies) which left me feeling as if a rug had been pulled from under my feet. Some years on, I still feel that I fall down just as hard, but it doesn't take me quite as long to get up again. However, the pain never completely goes away, the sharp pain being somewhat replaced by an ache of disappointment and deep sadness.

My own burnout at work and feelings of isolation from Barry contributed to the deterioration of our relationship, putting a deep strain on our marriage.

Barry

I assumed that I wouldn't automatically have children, which was possibly an unconscious strategy to protect myself from pain and disappointment if I didn't get married and if children didn't come along.

However, I was unprepared for the pain that Rosemary felt when it became clear that we may not have children. I felt inadequate, helpless and guilty, which meant that I didn't know what to say. The fear of saying the wrong thing meant that I didn't communicate, and I became afraid to ask Rosemary how she felt because I couldn't handle the painful responses. Mixed with my own burnout at work and at church, this isolated me from Rosemary.

Although I didn't handle the situation well, Rosemary testifies that I did some helpful things too. I didn't walk out, which would have been an escape from the pain. I tried to look at the situation through Rosemary's eyes in order to try and understand better, even though it was difficult for me to demonstrate empathy. I tried to remember to hug and hold Rosemary and allowed her to cry with me, which was essential for her.

b. What effects did infertility and our responses to it have on our marriage and other aspects of our lives?

We have mentioned some of the responses to infertility that culminated in Barry and Rosemary twice considering separation. In addition to this there were other effects. The following list includes some examples from our marriage but there will also be others that you may think of.

Church life:
We attend a large, active church where there are lots of families. We have at times felt very isolated. Friendships have been lost due to the change in others' circumstances and our struggle to maintain contact with friends who have become new parents.

Relationships with our families, friends and acquaintances:
We have been fortunate to have supportive parents and other family who have put no pressure on us and verbalise no expectations about children. However, we have had some highly unhelpful comments from acquaintances, as described in the prologue of this book.

Work:
Having got married, Rosemary didn't expect to still be employed throughout her working life. She has never been a career woman, which has made the whole concept of continuing to work very difficult. Starting a new job always brings mixed feelings as this is

a very tangible reminder of our infertility. She has also found it particularly hard seeing colleagues leaving work to have children.

Sex life:
The pressure on our sex life increased as we tried to conceive, which meant that this aspect of our relationship suffered a great deal. Times of romance diminished and sex became more mechanical, as we lost the perspective that God intends sex to be enjoyed for its own sake. Instead, it became only a tool to attempt procreation.

Identity:
Each person can mistakenly try to find their identity principally in anything other than as God's child. In Rosemary's case it was an attempt to try and find her identity as a mother, which led to deep disappointment as it became clear that we couldn't have children. We will discuss this further in chapter 4.

Post-childbearing years:
At the time of writing this resource, the impact of infertility through the menopause and beyond are not yet issues that have faced us. A number of feelings may arise in post-childbearing years for infertile couples; you may be in this position and have experienced other effects that are different from the examples given below:

- Going through the menopause may be particularly difficult, since it may engender feelings of finality regarding any possibility of having children.
- Fresh grief may be experienced as peers who have children speak of any milestones achieved by their offspring (for example, leaving school, passing a driving test, university entrance, setting up home, getting married).
- A particularly difficult experience may be seeing peers become grandparents.
- Loneliness may be experienced, particularly upon the death of one spouse. It is important for infertile couples to be part of a wider community, particularly a church family, in order to receive support and encouragement.
- Resentment at the need to continue with a career may be evident.

c. What principles can we identify from our responses to and the effects of infertility?

Many different and complex feelings can accompany infertility

For example:
Anger:
This may be expressed or concealed depending on the individual temperament.

Guilt:
This may be a particularly strong emotion for the spouse with whom the physical cause of infertility may lay; although general feelings of guilt at not fulfilling expectations of self and others may be equally powerful.

Isolation:
Feelings of isolation from contemporaries who are having children can occur. This impacts on the dynamics of relationships with others.

Disappointment:
May be felt with self, spouse, God or others. Rosemary describes this disappointment as a broken dream.

Sadness:
This can feel like an ache, particularly with the passage of time.

Incompleteness:
Rosemary has experienced a deep sense of feeling incomplete without children.

Effects on the marriage for better or worse

We both demonstrated healthy and unhealthy responses to infertility, which affected the strength of our marriage. Such responses (particularly in the early days) combined with the feelings described above and uncertainty about the future can affect whether or not a marriage will survive. Key to survival is an understanding by each spouse of how the other feels, which requires honest, frequent and open communication. In chapter 4 we will move from looking at the effects of infertility on marriages to looking at the effects on relationships with God.

There are practical things that we can do for one another because of agape love

The New Testament was originally written in Greek, and there are several different Greek words for our English word 'love'. Each of these words conveys different aspects of love, all of which are important in a marriage. *Eros* speaks of physical affinity and *philia* speaks of psychological affinity.

The third Greek word for love, *agape,* is a decision to meet another person's needs. *Agape* love is not an emotion dependent on either sexual or intellectual attraction. *Agape* love is practical love, love in action. It is the antithesis of selfishness. *Agape* love is not 'because of' but 'in spite of'. It makes no requirement of the object of its love. *Agape* love is demonstrated by investing resources in another person's well-being.

Agape love is also the mark of a Christian. God's goal for every believer is that we develop the character of Christ. The primary character quality emphasised in the Bible is love. The word 'love' in verses such as Matthew 22:37 and 39, Luke 6:27, Ephesians 5:25 is based on the root of *agape* in the original Greek. The fact that *agape* love is commanded should encourage us to know that it is possible.

In our marriage, we demonstrated *agape* love towards one another. Neither of us felt in love during our early struggles with infertility, but we were able to demonstrate *agape* love by investing our resources in the well-being of each other. Simple examples included making a cup of tea, preparing a meal, remembering to buy milk on the way home or running a bath.

Infertility affects marriages in a variety of ways

We have described some of the effects of infertility on our own marriage. There may be common effects for most marriages but each individual will also respond in their own unique way.

d. What does the Bible say about the pain of infertility?

The pain of not having children is rightly understood against the background of the importance placed upon children in the Bible, for example, Psalm 127:3–5:

Sons are a heritage from the LORD, children a reward from him. Like arrows in the hands of a warrior, are sons born in one's youth. Blessed is the man whose quiver is full of them.

Children in the Old Testament are portrayed as a sign of God's blessing, compared to the shame of not having children. As well as practical reasons, such as reliance on children in old age and to aid the family's economy, childbearing was important in ancient Israel because:

- Childbearing was the first commandment from God (Genesis 1:28).
- Procreation was linked to God's promises to Abraham (for example, Genesis 15:5).
- It was thought that childbearing was part of God's redemptive purpose, including the birth of Jesus.

Given this background, it makes sense that infertility will be associated with pain; and we see the pain of infertility in Scripture. Infertility is mentioned a number of times in both the Old and New Testaments. For example, Proverbs 30:15–16 lists four things that are never satisfied, one of which is the 'barren womb'.

It is important at this point to recognize that there are several Old Testament examples of God enabling barren women to conceive as part of his dealings with his people, Israel. If we do not understand these occurrences within the wider principles of Scripture we can easily and mistakenly equate infertility with a lack of faith.

e. What does the Bible say to someone who feels guilty over infertility?

The Bible's view of children (as set out above) could easily make an infertile couple feel guilty for not having children. However, it is important to explore what the Bible as a whole says about children and infertility.

Is procreation a requirement?

Genesis 1 affirms that procreation is a blessing given by God (verse 28) but does not declare this to be the primary purpose of marriage. Neither is a command for procreation seen in Genesis 2. However, the meaning of the term 'helper' in Genesis 2:18 and

20 suggests that the purpose of marriage is joint service of God in a relationship of loving companionship. Genesis 1:28 is probably best understood as a blessing and general intention for humankind rather than a command and a duty. Children are a gift from God, not a divine requirement. We therefore need not feel guilty if we have been unable to have children. If we, as infertile couples, do not share in Genesis 1:28, we are not receiving that particular blessing. This is why infertility is painful but we cannot link the associated pain with a lack of faith. A correct understanding of Scripture does not eliminate suffering.

Since children are not a divine requirement, we have often wondered if the words used in the Anglican marriage service could sound presumptuous:

> *The gift of marriage brings husband and wife together in the delight and tenderness of sexual union and joyful commitment to the end of their lives. It is given as the foundation of family life in which children are [born and] nurtured..... May they nurture their family with devotion, see their children grow in body, mind and spirit.*[3]

We have often stood together during weddings conducted in Anglican churches and found it painful to listen to these words. What should be a happy occasion becomes enormously difficult as we brace ourselves to hear these words, squeeze each other's hands as they are read, and then feel isolated and bereft. We wonder if these words could reinforce the unfortunate expectation that children will always follow after marriage.

Is infertility a punishment for sin?

Genesis 3 lists the results of human sin, with spiritual and physical consequences. Infertility isn't mentioned explicitly but the process of procreation is cursed (verse 16). Infertility should therefore be understood as a consequence of the fall.

God does punish disobedience with barrenness (for example, Genesis 20:17–18, Hosea 9:11) but such texts do not make a direct connection between infertility and individual sin. Luke gives a

[3] See details of the Anglican marriage service on the Church of England website: http://www.cofe.anglican.org/worship/liturgy/commonworship/texts/marriage/marriage.html

good example in his gospel (Luke 1:6–7). Elizabeth and Zechariah are described as 'upright in the sight of God', yet Elizabeth was barren.

What is your perspective on suffering?

There is no doubt that infertility causes great suffering. We have experienced feelings of isolation, loneliness, love towards a child that cannot be given, anger, anxiety and despair. Yet the Bible speaks often about our suffering as Christians.

We should not be surprised when we suffer (for example, 1 Peter 4:12) and we are told that our way into God's kingdom is marked by suffering (for example, Acts 14:22). The fall has affected our lives in every way, including fertility; and God uses suffering to produce patience, endurance and genuine faith (for example, James 1:2, Hebrews 10:35–6, 1 Peter 1:6). In trials like infertility, we follow Jesus who experienced great suffering and warned us of tribulation (for example, John 16:33).

Our desire here has not been to encourage you to ignore your pain or to try and be super-spiritual. However, we want to bring to your attention the teaching of the New Testament and encourage you to study Scripture for yourselves in order to formulate a sound theology of suffering within which you can begin to come to terms with your own infertility. As Christians we are called to suffer and should not be surprised if it happens. For us, one way in which the Lord has called us to suffer is through infertility. We would rather not have been through this but can see how God has developed endurance in us and gained glory for himself as a result.

f. Points for reflection

The aim of the following exercise is to help you look at how painful infertility is for you. Emotional pain is impossible to measure but it may be helpful to mark your responses to the questions and reflect upon them. By sharing your responses with your spouse it may give them fresh insights into your pain.

Please spend some time looking at the following questions on your own. When you have finished them, we suggest that you come back together with your spouse and discuss your answers.

We suggest that you give instant 'gut feeling' responses to questions 1–3 and spend no more than a minute or two on them.

Our responses to infertility, feelings and the effects

Questions 4-7 should take no longer than 15–20 minutes in total.

Some people may find it easier to express how they feel through drawing, painting or some other creative activity. If this works better for you, you could, for example, draw or paint how your infertility makes you feel, rather than writing about it. You could keep your work in a journal; and you may wish to talk through your work with your spouse.

Questions 1–3: Mark on the line below where you see yourself and your spouse at the present time. There are no right or wrong answers.

1. The pain of infertility feels:

As bad as it could feel *Barely noticeable*

____

2. My spouse:

Clearly knows how I feel *Barely knows how I feel*

____

3. I think that I:

Know clearly how my spouse feels *Barely know how my spouse feels*

____

4. Write here any words that describe how you feel about your infertility (maximum of five):

5. *List up to three things that your spouse does that is helpful for you as you try to cope with your infertility.*

6. *Is there anything unhelpful that your spouse does, which needs to be discussed?*

7. *Is there anything helpful your spouse could be doing for you that you need to raise with them?*

8. *How has your infertility affected other areas of your life, for example, church life, sex life, relationships with friends and family, identity, etc.?*

3. Grief

a. Rosemary's perspective on grief

During the process of trying to come to terms with our infertility, a turning point came for me when a friend in similar circumstances wisely explained that coping with infertility involves a grieving process. This was helpful because it made me realise that it was OK to cry and to feel so desperate at times. Until then I had often felt guilty for finding infertility so hard to cope with and I used to give myself a hard time when I broke down.

Grief associated with infertility does not follow a typical pattern. This is because we grieve for something that we have never had and there is fresh grief with each monthly cycle. In the early years of our infertility I described this as a monthly roller coaster ride, with the up of hope and the dreadful plunge back down to earth as the disappointment set in once again. Even now it is hard to let go of the hope completely. I still have all the hormones, the maternal instincts and a body designed to carry children. Sometimes I have personified my hormones and feel that they are screaming at me – they are a monthly reminder of what I don't have and yet for which I am biologically designed.

The grief of infertility is particularly hard to bear because there is no opportunity to say goodbye – no funeral, no line in the sand to demarcate a life that has come to an end. It was suggested to us by some wise counsellors that we consider holding a funeral for the children we weren't able to have. At first I recoiled from this idea completely – it seemed a dreadful and bizarre thing to do – something I couldn't entertain doing at all. Over time, however, after much discussion with Barry and prayer, we came to the point of deciding it would be helpful to hold a funeral. It gave us the opportunity to say goodbye. We decided to write a letter to our children, telling them that we love them, miss them and describing how we would have hoped to care for and nurture them. The letter closed with us giving them to God. We then went to Lindisfarne – a place chosen not primarily because of its Christian associations but because it is several hundred miles from where we live. It is also an isolated place because the road access is via a tidal causeway. When the tide comes in, Lindisfarne becomes an island. It is hard to explain why this was important to us – but we wanted a sense of being cut off during the funeral. I read our letter to the children out loud, Barry prayed, we burned the letter and scattered the ashes as we looked out to sea from an ancient prayer hole. The symbolism was important to us and it gives us something to look back on, as a point in time when we said goodbye. Of course this is only one example – but it seemed to be the right one for us.

The following year we decided to pay to have a tree dedicated to the memory of the children. Although there is no visible plaque in the forest we chose, we have a card at home with the dedication words written on. I have found this helpful as it gives me something less painful than Lindisfarne to look back on as a way of remembering them. Perhaps parallels could be drawn between what we did and the funeral of a loved one followed by a subsequent thanksgiving service.

Writing this section has probably been the hardest part of putting this resource together. It is extraordinarily painful to see these words written down in black and white and to know that they are about Barry and me. We hope and pray that you have not felt them to be emotive in any unhelpful way. Our purpose in writing is not to tug at anyone's heart strings, but rather to share our experiences with the hope that reading them will be helpful for you as you cope with your own personal situations. We hope that our openness will help you to be open with one another and with God.

b. The unique nature of grief associated with infertility

Most of us have either known someone who has been bereaved, or have been bereaved ourselves. Some of us may also be aware of theories about the stages of grief, which can be useful in answering the common question 'how long will it last?' This is not the place to explore these theories and there are many books on the subject. However, like other forms of loss, the loss associated with infertility is unique, as is the grief associated with it.

Commonly accepted stages of grief [4]

Grief is often described in terms of a number of stages that people pass through. It is important to note that not everyone experiences each stage of grief, or they may experience some of the stages in a different order. It is not a neat, ordered process. Some people may feel that they are experiencing more than one of the stages at the same time. In other words, grief is messy.

Having said that, we thought it would be helpful to set out the stages identified in the process of loss and describe how we have experienced each stage during our journey through infertility.

SHOCK – possible numbness, fear, uncertainty and disorientation

We had begun to realise that there was a problem after the first few months of trying to conceive. The difficulties were a shock to us, although with our medical backgrounds, we had wondered about the impact of Barry's hernia repair. We also experienced a degree of shock when infertility was confirmed by our consultant, because it was hard to come to terms with the finality of the diagnosis.

DENIAL – hope that the loss is not real or may be rectified

Rosemary described earlier the influence of her monthly cycle, which makes denial more likely because of the hopes that remain month-to-month. After the final confirmation of our infertility and taking the decision not to adopt or pursue IVF, it is still hard to avoid denial whilst we are technically of reproductive age.

ANGER – can be directed at God, self, at that which has been lost or at those who caused the loss

Rosemary was not consciously angry with Barry because his need for a hernia repair was not his fault. However, there may have been subconscious anger about the infertility itself and Barry's inability to communicate. Both of us have been angry with God for different reasons, and it has been vital to

[4] See further: Griffiths, T., *Lost and then Found:* p15, Carlisle, 1999

remember that such feelings do not jeopardise our relationships with God. We see God's people in Scripture being very honest with him in expressing their feelings, such as Elijah, Jonah and the Psalmist.

GUILT – thinking, for example, 'did I cause the loss?' or 'could I have prevented it?'

Barry has experienced significant feelings of guilt. He knows intellectually that he had not set out to hurt Rosemary through not being able to father children, but it is very hard knowing that he has hurt her, albeit unwittingly. It is important to him that Rosemary frequently provides reassurance of her understanding of this and her acceptance of him. Men can be fragile emotionally and easily broken. Barry has experienced this brokenness during the difficult times in our marriage.

BARGAINING – attempting to restore the loss, maybe by bargaining with God

Rosemary didn't attempt any sort of bargaining either with God or herself. It would have been understandable if she had said things to God along the lines of, 'I'll be the best mother in the world if you give me children', but she can honestly say that she never had these thoughts.

Barry by contrast found that dark and persistent thoughts came frequently to him, with images of possible problems associated with having children. These included images of a sick or delinquent child, and images of disunity with Rosemary caused by having children. It was as if he was subconsciously rationalising why it would be good NOT to have children. He was bargaining with himself.

DEPRESSION – leading to feelings of hopelessness, meaninglessness, powerlessness

Clinical depression is an illness and can be difficult to diagnose. It is often confused by non-medical people with *feeling down* or *depressed,* which can be very different and is not an illness. Looking back, we can both recognise periods of time when one or other of us has felt depressed. We are aware that other life events may be very difficult to cope with; for example, Rosemary going through the menopause, close friends/family becoming grandparents, our godchildren having children of their own. These events could cause depression or depressed feelings.

ACCEPTANCE – in spite of the loss, a realisation that life can continue. Acceptance doesn't erase the memories

Acceptance can be very difficult with infertility, in comparison with some other forms of loss. Many other losses relate to a single event that is conspicuous; for example, seeing the dead body of a loved one. Although most of us have not seen God resurrecting the dead (!), he *could* perform a miracle and allow a pregnancy for us. We have found it very difficult to get *closure* on our grief, and this is compounded by regular exposure to pregnant women and young families.

In extreme cases, some infertile people feel their loss to such an extent that self-harm or suicide is possible. It is vital for couples coping with infertility to acknowledge that they are going through a grieving process. This grief may manifest itself in a number of ways and needs to be worked through as much as possible. As Rosemary has written, this was a major step forward for us and has allowed us to understand much more what is happening in our thoughts, emotions and reactions.

c. Coping with grief

Each of us can respond to loss in different ways. Some of our attitudes can be constructive, whereas others can be destructive. Here are some attitudes that could be experienced during the grieving process.[5] We may demonstrate a mixture of these responses with varying degrees of intensity, and these may vary from day-to-day. You may identify with these attitudes completely, partly or not at all, depending on the stage of your journey:

Constructive attitudes may include:

Accepting what has happened
Hopefulness
Faith in the future

[5] Richardson, J., *A Death in the Family*: p38, Oxford, 1993

Making the most of what is left
Willingness to recover
Being thankful for the past
Accepting help and friendship
Committing everything to God

Destructive attitudes may include:

Bitterness
Despair
Pride
Shutting yourself away
Self-pity
Looking for someone to blame
Becoming a martyr
Cursing God

We have found that it is easy to adopt the destructive attitudes and hard to adopt the constructive ones! For example, we have described above how hard it is to accept what has happened, and to have faith in the future. By contrast, self-pity, becoming a martyr and cursing God are remarkably easy to slip into. We have been learning on our journey that it is our *responsibility* to be willing to recover (this may feel radical) and to commit everything to God. Committing everything to God is an issue of trust and depends on our relationships with him. This is particularly challenging and is the subject of the next chapter.

Many counsellors agree that emotions are generally safer when they are expressed, rather than being internalised. Acknowledgement and expression of grief are painful, but this doesn't mean that we shouldn't do both. Perhaps you could ask some close friends/family to pray for you as you try to do this.

d. What does the Bible say about grief?

We see in John 11:17–37 that Jesus grieved for his friend Lazarus and showed compassion in ministering to Mary and Martha in their grief. This compassion was extended by Jesus to many others, such as the widow who lost her son in Luke 7:11–17, and to his own disciples who would grieve for him as his sacrificial death on the cross approached (John 16:16–24). The fact that God the Son could grieve and had compassion upon grieving people legitimises our grief.

During our time with some wise counsellors we studied the account of the death of King David's illegitimate son in 2 Samuel 12:13–23. God struck the child that was born of David's adulterous relationship with Bathsheba and a contrite and repentant David asked God to spare the child during the following week through fasting and prayer. Yet he had been told by the prophet Nathan that the child would die, so whilst maintaining hope that God may relent and spare the child, perhaps David had expressed his grief in advance, as it were. When the child died, David, surprisingly, drew a line under his grief and moved on. He was of course devastated, but content that God had acted rightly. David *accepted* God's decision.

We have found it hard to *accept* God's decision about our infertility. Yet David's striking response, where we see him continuing to walk in God's ways, demonstrates that it must be possible to accept God's will in such a painful matter. David models grief to us and he is not condemned by God for it. It would be reasonable to suspect that for the rest of his life, David lamented deeply the loss of his child, but he did move on with his life.

e. Points for reflection

The aim of the following exercise is to help you to apply some of the information about grief to your own situation of infertility. You will be able to compare your grief with that of Rosemary and Barry, consider your stage of grief, and any potentially constructive or destructive attitudes.

Depending on the stage of your journey, you may wish to read these questions and let them sink in before coming back to answer them. Don't be afraid to wait until either or both of you are ready to discuss them. When you do, spend about 30–45 minutes working through them individually before coming together to discuss your answers.

1. Did you realise that grief tends to accompany infertility? How does this make you feel?

2. What, if anything, do you identify with as you read Rosemary's account of her grief? Is there anything that you don't identify with?

3. List any feelings/emotions that you have experienced, which Rosemary didn't describe of herself?

4. How appropriate would it be in your own marriage to hold a funeral for the children you haven't had? List the reasons for your response.

5. Looking at the common stages of grief, at which stage:

a. Might you be at right now?

b. Might your spouse be at right now?

Try to think about what led you to these conclusions.

6a. Try to list the *constructive* attitudes that you have in relation to your infertility.

6b. Now list the *destructive* attitudes that you have held or to which you are prone.

7a. How could your spouse support you at the moment with your grief?

7b. How might you support your spouse with their grief?

7c. How might you help yourself?

8. How does the example of David's grief (2 Samuel 12:13–23) make you feel?

9. Is there anything practical that you could set time aside to do in order to express your grief?

Think about how your culture expresses grief. In British culture, grief may not be expressed as openly as in some other cultures. Ideas for expressing grief may include drawing, painting, poetry, walking in the park to kick leaves, throwing stones into the sea, allowing time in front of an open fire to sit and weep. You may be able to think of others.

4. Infertility and our individual relationships with God

Our relationships within marriage and with other people can be profoundly affected by infertility. But what about our individual relationships with God? In this section we will describe how our relationships with God were affected. We will then invite you to think this through for yourselves.

a. What effect did infertility have on our individual relationships with God?

Rosemary

As it became clear that we may not have children, my relationship with God deteriorated. We mentioned earlier my anger which was not expressed in an open relationship with my heavenly father, possibly because it didn't feel safe to do so. In fact, I couldn't talk to God about infertility and couldn't pray for myself. The additional confusion about the future direction of my life, for example, in terms of career, made it hard for me to trust God.

Looking back to that time of intense, raw pain, I am able to see the danger of trying to find my identity as a mother, which perhaps I felt subconsciously would define me as a woman. I found it hard to maintain an eternal perspective, particularly when feeling surrounded by others who have children. This difficulty is understandable given the pain of my immediate situation.

Barry

In contrast to Rosemary, I constantly talked to God about our infertility, asking for his will to be done. This may have been easier because I felt more ambivalent about having children. My pain of seeing Rosemary's struggle led me to become angry with God, but this was expressed fully in prayer. I found Rosemary's lack of communication with God very difficult.

I too struggled with an issue around identity. This was because my identity was found more in serving God than in being in relationship with God. I was convinced that not having children was a testimony to God's sovereignty – in other words I believed that God was deliberately not calling Rosemary and me to be parents. I remain convinced that God is in control of our circumstances but have struggled to cope with the pain associated with it. My weakness has been to desire freedom from the pain more than desiring a close and intimate relationship with God.

b. What principles do our responses illustrate?

Different relationships with God

Each of our responses to God was very different. It is important to be aware of how good or bad our relationship with God has been and to be honest about how much or little we are able to trust him. If trust is difficult (which is very understandable), then open and honest dialogue with God is essential. He knows our thoughts anyway! (See Psalm 139, particularly verse 2).

God desires to be the head of each marriage and this can be more difficult if either spouse is struggling in their relationship with God. This can also lead to husband and wife being out of step with each other spiritually.

c. What can we say about the issue of identity?

There is a Christian counselling model that refers to crucial longings deep down in every person for *security, self-worth* and *significance.*[6] The model suggests that these crucial longings are intended to be met by God in the following ways:

- Having a sense of *security* through the knowledge that he loves us unconditionally.
- Knowing that he values us which gives us a sense of *self-worth.*
- Finding our *significance* in being God's children. It can be helpful in our Christian walk to remember that God is our heavenly father.

[6] A basic overview of this counselling model can be found in chapter 6 of Sheldon, M., Ames, D., *To Bind up the Broken Hearted,* Guildford, 1999

How we are perceived by others, whilst important to us, should not be as important as God's view of us.

Security, *self-worth* and *significance* contribute to our sense of identity, which includes different aspects to our lives; for example, the gifts that God has given us and what we do with them. However, the principal aspect of our identity is as children of God. The language of the New Testament, for example, in passages such as John 1:12–13, Romans 8:12–17, Ephesians 1 and 1 John 3:1–3 reminds us that those of us who trust Christ for salvation are identified as God's children. This should give us a sense of identity and purpose in our earthly lives as well as confidence for eternity, since our identity as children of God means that we are welcomed into an everlasting relationship with him.

Since the fall of man, however, all people have rebelled against God, which leaves us prone to seeking security, self-worth, significance and therefore identity elsewhere. For example, some find their principal identity in their job, their financial status, or a human relationship. These things are important but can become idols if they become more important in our lives than God himself.

Jeremiah 2:4–13 illustrates how Israel forsook God and followed 'worthless idols' instead. God describes himself in verse 13 as 'the spring of living water' and declares that his people have forsaken him and instead have dug 'broken cisterns that cannot hold water'. This means that instead of letting God meet all their needs, illustrated by him being a 'spring of living water', Israel tried to obtain their own *water* supply by digging *leaky wells*. In other words, Israel attempted to find satisfaction for their crucial needs elsewhere apart from God. Although originally directed at Israel, it is surely reasonable to apply these words to ourselves. Seeking our principal identity in anything other than God today is still like digging a 'broken cistern'.

Painful as infertility is, our responses that you read about earlier suggest that being children of God had not been the principal source of our identity as people, but rather other things had taken precedence, including having children. Such tendencies are a risk in all people but are not surprising, possibly because of the immediate feelings that our human needs arouse in us compared with a feeling of intangibility about eternity with God that is promised to all Christians. Therefore the tangible pain of infertility may make it feel that having children *is* essential, which we saw earlier may be exacerbated in the Anglican marriage service and is powerfully seen in the family life of most married couples that surround us.

However, it is important to check the Bible to see if God sees children as essential.

The Book of Isaiah suggests that infertility isn't the worst of calamities, or that it has to be overcome in order to participate in the purpose of God and experience true joy:

> *'Sing, O barren woman, you who never bore a child; burst into song, shout for joy, you who were never in labour; because more are the children of the desolate woman than of her who has a husband,' says the* LORD. *(Isaiah 54:1. See also Isaiah 56:4–5)*

Having children doesn't necessarily signify God's favour or merit any spiritual reward. Instead, the barrier between us and God comes when we fail to put our trust in him for our salvation. Our principal identity is as children of God.

d. Where does faith fit in?

We have been fortunate that no one has told us that 'we would have children if only we had more faith'. The danger of such thinking is that it is human-centred rather than God-centred. God calls us in Scripture to have faith and he allows us the privilege of praying for things to happen. However, prayer must always be according to God's will and Jesus models this in his prayer in the Garden of Gethsemane, *Father, if you are willing, take this cup from me; yet not my will, but yours be done* (Luke 22:42). We must be prepared for God to know what is best for us and for him to answer our prayers according to his will. If we think that having children is a matter of having enough faith on its own without remembering God's prerogative to answer as he wishes, we could fall into the trap of relying on our human ability to have faith, rather than on the sovereignty of God. The danger of this trap is not only an inherently incorrect view of God, but it may induce crippling guilt.

e. Points for reflection

The aim of these questions is to help you think about how you feel about God in relation to your infertility. If you can articulate your feelings about God, it may help you to express those feelings towards him in prayer. It may also help you to describe your feelings to your spouse, leading to a deeper shared understanding.

You may wish to set aside some time and space to look through these questions on your own, which could mean going for a walk to meditate upon them, or sitting in a comfortable chair with pen and paper. Try setting aside 30–45 minutes in the first instance. When you have finished them, we suggest that you come back together and discuss your answers.

1. As you think of your own situation of infertility, to what extent do you identify with either Rosemary or Barry's responses to God that you have read about?

2. How does the biblical material discussed in this session make you feel towards God?

3. How easy is it to pray for yourself, your infertility and coping with it?

4. What prayers would be helpful to pray?

5. How can you encourage your spouse in their walk with God?

6. How could your spouse encourage you in your walk with God?

5. Moving forward

In this section we will explore two main issues.

First, we will look at the issue of our individual relationships with God and his headship of our own family (we are convinced that the two of us are legitimately defined as a *family*). We hope to suggest some biblical approaches to considering the most important relationship that each of us will have, in order that we can invest in it and work slowly towards finding our security, self-worth and significance in God.

Second, we will share something of our experience of trying to move forward in a practical sense. The aim is for you to discuss how these ideas may help you in your own marriage, or stimulate you to come up with other ideas.

a. Moving forward in our relationships with God

Bible truths are important but infertility still hurts!

Important and familiar as the biblical truths we have been reading about may be, at times they seem to make the pain worse rather than better. This has certainly been our experience. Anyone in pain, including couples struggling with infertility, desperately want to be healed of the pain and to live lives for God, but his other blessings seem to be a second best or a consolation prize particularly if we feel that he has denied us children. There are no trade-offs and we have sometimes felt resentful of our current circumstances. For example, with children, it would not have been possible for the two of us to go to Bible college – but that doesn't take away the pain. Our biblical studies have been fantastic, but it feels like a high price to pay.

It is understandable to feel angry and frustrated with God, particularly if we feel that we would make good parents and would be able to provide a good home and model Christ to our children. It just doesn't make sense. How then, can biblical truths about infertility help us rather than send us into despair? Here are some ideas:

i. Read about infertile people in the Bible

We read from the accounts of women like Sarah (Genesis 11–21) and Hannah (1 Samuel 1–2) of great despair in infertility. It is vital to read these as historical accounts and to consciously remember that the God who was with those women and was sovereign over their infertility is the same God who listens to your prayers now. This does not necessarily mean that he will restore fertility, but it can be helpful to remember that each of our family situations has been decided by God and is not a random occurrence. We also see from women such as these that God's provision of children is for HIS purpose and not theirs, because the majority of children eventually born to barren women are important figures in Israelite history. Examples include Isaac, Jacob, Joseph, Samson, Samuel and John the Baptist. Even Christ's lineage is traced through unexpected births to barren women. See Christ's genealogy in Matthew 1:1–17.

ii. Remember the role of prayer

Christians believe that God answers prayer, but many secretly believe also that God won't answer *their* particular prayer. This can mean that individual Christians don't really pray for themselves. Prayer to God for children is seen in passages like Genesis 20 and Luke 1. Therefore, praying to be able to have children is a completely legitimate thing to do yourself and to ask others to do for you.

However, we have to pray in line with God's will and be ready to accept and obey God's answer.

Rosemary finds it comparatively easy to pray for others, but finds it very hard to pray for herself – and it's even more difficult when feeling angry towards God. In contrast Barry finds it much easier to pray for himself.

Both of us have at times succumbed to *demanding* from God rather than *asking*; and also of wanting God's gifts more than relationship with God himself. This is not to say that the reason for our infertility is linked to this, but this issue has identified our true priorities. Of course, you may be able to say that you do want relationship with God desperately – you just want children as well! There are no easy answers to this, except to say that honesty in prayer is vital, which may include crying out to him, telling him all that you feel – even expressing deep hostility towards him. We must remember that he knows our thoughts and feelings. The Psalms may help us cry to God in prayer; as do the historical accounts of barren women as we identify with them and imagine ourselves in their situations, perhaps praying as they did. How did they pray? Well, for Zechariah and Elizabeth to be called 'upright in the sight of God' (Luke 1:6), their prayers for children (Luke 1:13) must have been godly. This begs the question 'what is godly prayer or a godly attitude?' Perhaps God's rebuke to Job (Job 38–42) for demanding vindication illustrates that we can and should express our hopes, desires and pain, but never a *demand* to God for anything.

iii. Remember the role of faith

We need to be careful with accounts such as Elizabeth in Luke 1. This could easily be interpreted by thinking that if we have enough faith or pray enough, God will give us children. As has been described earlier, we have not been on the receiving end of well-meaning Christians who doubt our faith because we don't have children. However we would guess that at least some readers may have experienced this, which is unhelpful and untrue. Instead, we could consider the following questions as they apply to our marriages and to us as individuals:

- What is God trying to teach us through this?
- What does God want to do in our lives through this?
- Instead of asking 'why me/us, Lord?', try asking 'why NOT me/us Lord?'

We are called to have faith in God and to present our requests to him. However, Hebrews 11:39 speaks of faithful servants who are commended for their faith but did not receive what was promised. Faith means believing in a loving and sovereign God and trusting him for his answer. This is costly, because it means yielding to God and accepting his decision for our infertility. This doesn't contradict what we said earlier, namely that it is acceptable to pray for children. We just need to bring prayer and faith together by adding to the end of our prayers 'your will be done'. There is the danger of wanting healing and protection more than wanting God himself and to serve him, particularly as we live in a culture that demands the absence of pain and immediate healing. As God's children we can be sure that he is sovereign over our lives and that he loves us. He wants us to make him a higher priority than having children or even healing from our feelings of pain this side of heaven. This is because he claims to be more valuable to us than anything else and has promised us an eternity, the joy of which we cannot currently comprehend (1 Corinthians 2:9). We can and should test these claims by reading the Bible and getting to know God better through it.

b. Moving forward in practical ways

Our own experience of trying to move forward has been difficult because:

- There are constant reminders of children around us and we are more sensitive to them; for example, parents pushing buggies (there always seem to be hundreds of them) plus heavily pregnant women!
- It is hard to maintain an eternal perspective in our materialistic, western culture.
- It is hard to maintain an eternal perspective when we are in pain and the here and now fills our horizons.
- It is hard to trust God for the future. Sometimes it feels like God answers prayer, but not our prayers, in the way we want.

Some practical thoughts follow about moving forward. Some of these may be very hard to read and may not be appropriate for you or quite right for where you are at now. Even if this is the case, we hope that as you persevere on your journey, you will revisit these ideas and prayerfully consider them as possibilities for the future.

i. Acknowledge the pain

Looking at Scripture as a whole, it is reasonable to conclude that God's general intention for married couples is to have children. It therefore makes sense that not having children will lead to pain. It can be very hard, for example, to live as a woman in a body that is designed to carry children. Our society and even some of our churches deny or ignore pain such as this.

Consider couples who have been bereaved of a child. To some extent, society and churches enter into and share the pain of those couples. It is harder for society and churches to relate to the loss of not having had a child at all, but it is still a bereavement. Infertility is a silent and unseen issue – people don't know by looking at the two of us that we cannot have children.

We should learn or continue to be real about our pain. We need to give ourselves permission to hurt, but it is difficult because infertility seems to be a taboo subject in church; in some ways understandably so as it is emotive and very personal to each couple.

ii. Express yourself in healthy ways

As we indicated earlier, counsellors often say that 'emotions are safer when they are expressed', but the expression of emotions needs to be done as healthily as possible. We have already given some ideas in the points for reflection within each chapter. Neither of us is especially creative in expressing ourselves and practical crafts such as using clay, collage and sketch tend not to appeal to us. However, if creative methods appeal more to you, please consider how you could use these.

Here are some other ideas:

- Find some Psalms where you can identify with the Psalmist's emotions, which include anger and disappointment. You may like to re-read these Psalms and consider using them as a means of expressing yourself to God. It's worth noting that recent biblical scholarship has emphasised that this is the most important way of using and understanding the Psalms, instead of focusing merely on their original historical context.
- Write a letter to God, expressing your deepest feelings towards him. Try reading the letter out loud to him as a prayer.
- Write a poem which could be addressed to God, to the children you never had, your spouse, or to anybody else important to you.
- Keep a journal. A journal may mean a diary of thoughts, feelings and milestones. You can write in your journal as much or as little as you like. Journals can be particularly helpful over time to look back on and see how your journey has progressed and how you have changed. Journals can sound unappealing

because people may think that they need to write well or often. This is not the case. A journal is very personal and we would recommend starting small. This may mean trying to write a few sentences once a month or once a week, just to help you to get going.

iii. Remember some key, practical truths

- Our lives are very short.
- Infertility is NOT our eternity. We will not have to live with infertility for ever, but life with God is eternal for the believer.
- Life will not always be like this – we will have fuller lives in heaven than we have on earth, even with children.

iv. Take reasonable care of ourselves

Think of practical things that you can do to protect yourselves from unnecessary reminders. Examples include not going to the morning service at church on mothers' day if your church particularly celebrates this, or watching out for well-intentioned requests to be godparents if you suspect that there is an element of pity in the request that could lead to difficulties later. Don't be afraid to say 'no thanks' if a well-intentioned friend asks if you want to hold their baby.

Learning to deal with unhelpful comments from others who do not understand the issues around infertility is valuable. This may involve challenging people by highlighting to them that their enquiries may cause us hurt. If we don't feel strong enough to challenge unhelpful comments, the easier but unwise option may be to internalise our responses. Unhelpful comments are rarely intentional. However, comments can be thoughtless or even raise false hopes. Try not to dwell on them, even though this is difficult.

There is a danger of idealising parenthood. Remember that there are many parents in pain for a variety of reasons, for example, bereavement, illness, time pressures, or rebellion. Infertile couples may well say 'but I'd at least like to have had the opportunity!' Yet this doesn't change the essential truth that parenthood, like procreation, is tainted by the fall.

Try to avoid isolation within your marriage and from outsiders. Feeling isolated is a key drain on our strength. Do you each have people that you pray with regularly? This could be a prayer partner, a prayer triplet, or friends from a small group at church. Are you in contact with other couples with infertility?

v. Consider what infertility might mean for our service to God?

Prayerfully consider, with the counsel of others, your gifting and potential areas to serve. We can seek to serve God either in spite of infertility, or because of it. In our case, this involves the opportunity to undertake pastoral care, to study God's word and get to know him better. It is a tough call for the two of us to consider that not having children was the way into study and developing our relationships with God. We have been taught painfully that God's will for us is to desire him more than anything else. We are challenged in Scripture to seek and answer God's call.

Watch out for seeing God's plan for our lives without children as a second best, which breeds resentment and bitterness. Hard as it is to acknowledge, God's will for us is the best.

Be a witness to others in your pain. How can you model godly sorrow? Do you need to consider whether you are pursuing parenthood at any cost? Have you an eternal hope that is maintained in the storm of infertility?

c. Points for reflection

The aim of these questions is to help you to think about moving forward, as you consider our experiences and ideas from this chapter. Try to spend about 30–45 minutes thinking about the questions and then compare your thoughts with each other.

See if you can come up with an individual and a joint action plan. This could include short, medium and long-term goals. For example, think about something you could do soon, and something you could aim to do in the months ahead. What you do may be based on our suggestions or ideas that you come up with yourself.

As we said at the start of this book, we appreciate that your situation may feel very raw and you may not yet be ready to think about looking at the questions. This particularly applies to the questions in this section. It is important to give yourselves time to process your situation. Don't attempt to move forward too soon, but don't put it off indefinitely either. If you are not ready yet, perhaps you could consider making a note to return to these questions in a few weeks or months. We don't want to give the impression that by the time you read this section, you will automatically be ready to move on.

1. *How does the biblical material discussed in this section make you feel about God?*

2. *Might God be speaking to you about your relationship with him as you read this biblical material? If so, how?*

3. *Which of the suggested ways to move forward in our relationships with God are helpful for you at the moment? Which are not helpful at the moment?*

4. *Which of the practical suggestions are helpful for you at the moment? Which are not helpful at the moment?*

5. *What other ideas do you have about moving forward from where you are right now?*

Epilogue

We expect that it will have been painful to work through this resource, but our prayer is that it has been helpful and constructive. By telling our stories, establishing some principles and looking at the Bible, we have attempted to offer a framework for you to explore the effects of infertility on your relationships with God and with your spouse.

Having worked through this resource, you may wish to think about anything you would like to say to those listed below. This may be through prayer, in person, by letter, through writing poetry, painting a picture or by some other means that would be helpful for you. See also the ideas in the last section *Moving forward in practical ways.*

* *God*

* *Yourself*

* *Your spouse*

* *Close friends and family*

* *Your church leaders*

* *The children you haven't had*

About
Mission to Marriage & Christian Marriage Ministries
The UK's specialist marriage ministry

The charity was founded by Dave and Joyce Ames in the early 1970s. Since then it has helped thousands of couples and hundreds of churches with all sorts of issues through:

- Public enrichment events, helping couples not to take their marriage for granted;
- Church-based events, including helping churches to develop their own marriage ministry;
- Marriage preparation, helping engaged couples get off to a good start;
- Specialist training events for counselling organisations, Bible colleges and missionary organisations;
- Private counselling and consultations, helping individuals and couples address specific problems in their marriage.

If you've never come across us before, don't be surprised! We do little advertising as most of our work comes by recommendation.

If you think we might be able to help you in any way, or perhaps work with your church, please don't hesitate to get in contact. If it's about counselling we'll naturally treat your enquiry in strict confidence. The easiest way to find out more about us is via our website, where you'll also find details of our other resources: www.christianmarriageministries.co.uk – but you can also contact us via our registered office. The address is at the front of this book. Although it's in Wales we work all over the UK and abroad.

Dr Tony Hobbs,
Director